Free from Plantar Fasciitis Forever

Eliminate your
Foot and Heel Pain in
14 Days or Less

Free from Plantar Fasciitis Forever

Cover, Images, Photos, and Formatting by Jeong Da Jeong

1 in 10 people are estimated to be affected by plantar fasciitis during their lifetime.

Medical Disclaimer

The information in this book is not intended or implied to be a substitute for professional medical advice, diagnosis, or treatment. All content, including text, graphics, images, and information, contained on or available through this book is for general information purposes only.

The author makes no representation and assumes no responsibility for the accuracy of the information contained on or available through this book, and such information is subject to change without notice.

You are encouraged to confirm any information obtained from or through this book with other sources, and review all information regarding any medical advice or treatment with your physician.

I am not a doctor. I am sharing my personal experience with plantar fasciitis.

Never disregard professional medical advice or delay seeking medical treatment because of something you have read on or accessed through this book.

The author is neither responsible nor liable for any advice, course of treatment, diagnosis or any other information that you obtain through this book.

Preface

If you're reading this book, you likely suffer from plantar fasciitis. Now that we have identified the problem, we need a solution. I think I've got it.

I strongly believe, based on my own results and those of others who have followed the protocol outlined in this book, that you can be free from plantar fasciitis within weeks. I am going to repeat that: You should feel better in a matter of weeks from your very first day of following the protocol described in this book. I think there is no question as to whether you will improve. It is only a question of how fast you will improve.

I had a severe case of plantar fasciitis for 8 months. In addition to the long duration of pain, I had limited mobility because I suffered from bilateral plantar fasciitis which means both of my feet were affected.

The great news is that I eventually discovered how to eliminate my plantar fasciitis in only 14 days without drugs or expensive products or services.

To heal this quickly after so much frustration, I felt

compelled to write this book.

Table of Contents

Introduction

Insoles and arch supports; compression socks; foot taping; foot rollers; foot massage balls and tools; orthotic shoes; foot and leg braces; night splint boots; shock wave therapy; pain relief slippers; cold and warm therapy foot wraps; calf and foot stretchers; ointments and creams; supplements and drugs; steroid, botox, and plasma injections; surgery.

These are some of the products and treatments available for plantar fasciitis.

Notice that surgery was mentioned last on the list. That's because surgical treatment - plantar fasciotomy - tends to be the last resort to relieve plantar fasciitis pain.

But get this, I've read that it's not uncommon for people to be recommended surgery if their plantar fasciitis pain hasn't resolved after six months of conservative treatment.

Yikes!

I suffered from plantar fasciitis for 8 months. That means had I visited a medical clinic then, I could have been encouraged to undergo surgery, which certainly is not without risks. Plantar fasciotomy complications include recurring heel pain, slow wound healing, and nerve tissue damage.

I rarely say yikes, but in this case, I think the word is appropriate. Because as you'll soon learn, I was able to eliminate my severe case of plantar fasciitis with a straightforward protocol which didn't involve expensive treatments and I most certainly didn't have surgery.

That is not to say I didn't try many techniques or products. In fact, I had tried so many plantar fasciitis exercises to no avail and suffered for so long that I was beginning to think that I wouldn't be able to walk again without pain, let alone run or jump rope or engage in many of the other forms of physical activity that typically fill much of my leisure time.

However, after months of frustration, I serendipitously made a connection between a feat I had previously accomplished - learning the middle splits - and how best to approach treating my plantar fasciitis.

And after just two weeks, I was able to walk, jump, and even run without pain. Actually, since I noticed signs of relief after just a few days into my new treatment plan, I felt so confident that I would quickly make a complete recovery, that I registered for a half-marathon that was taking place on St. Patrick's Day just 15 days away, despite not having run in almost one year.

As I crossed the finish line that day, I was tired, but I had no foot or heel pain whatsoever. Quite a remarkable achievement considering just a few weeks earlier simply walking was painstaking. How awesome!

As a lifelong sport and adventure enthusiast, I am no stranger to injuries. I've had dozens of blisters and stitches plus numerous fractured bones including toes, fingers, and ribs. One of my worst injuries was an ice hockey-related broken foot together with a ruptured Achilles tendon that sidelined me for several months and involved a cast, crutches, and at one point a wheelchair.

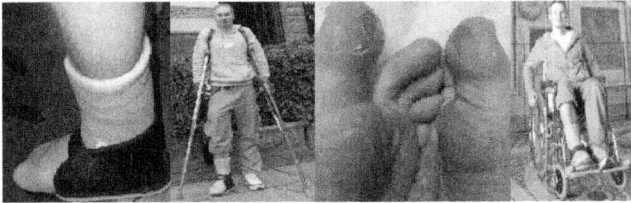

BUT nothing impacted my mobility over such a long period of time as plantar fasciitis.

I was so thrilled and relieved when I recovered from plantar fasciitis that I had to write this book and share what worked for me in the hope that the information can help you or someone you know avoid unnecessary pain or indeed a long layoff from a physical activity you enjoy or even your job if it demands you being physically active.

In the following chapters, I will cover the prevalence, symptoms, and risk factors for plantar fasciitis as well as the commonly prescribed exercises for treating plantar fasciitis. Then I will share the exact protocol I performed that enabled me to completely eliminate my severe case of bilateral plantar fasciitis in only 14 days.

The stretches and exercises in my protocol are the same ones I use to keep my plantar fasciitis from returning and therefore can be used to avoid plantar fasciitis in the first place.

As an addendum, I have included five additional exercises for increasing the strength and flexibility of the feet, ankle, and lower legs.

Plantar Fasciitis Prevalence, Symptoms, and Risk Factors

Let's briefly clarify what plantar fasciitis is in one sentence: Plantar fasciitis, pronounced plan-tar fa-shee-ai-tuhs, is one of the most common causes of heel and foot pain, specifically of the band of tissue that runs across the bottom of each foot and connects the heel bone to the base of the toes.

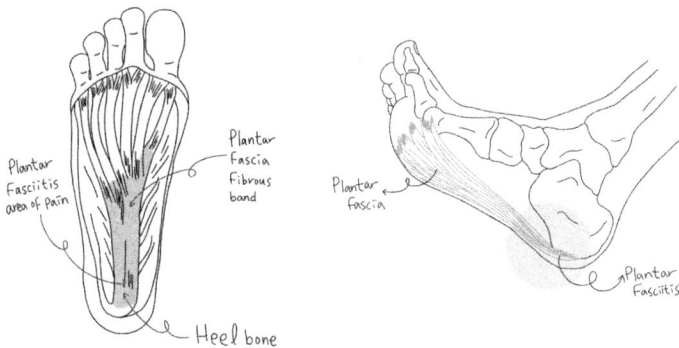

Plantar fasciitis pain is typically the worst when a person takes their first steps upon awakening from sleep, although long periods of standing can also trigger the pain. Standing up after sitting, especially when seated for prolonged periods can also result in immense pain. The pain can be so intense that it causes some people to sit back down after attempting to stand. I can attest to this. On several occasions, I couldn't stand up on my first attempt due to pain nor walk fast enough after standing in order to answer the phone or doorbell in time.

For many people, plantar fasciitis is unilateral, meaning it affects just one side of the body, that is, the left or right foot. However, it may present bilaterally in some cases. Unfortunately, I fell into that category, as I will explain shortly.

1 in 10 people are estimated to be affected by plantar fasciitis at some point during their lifetime.

Given that billions of dollars are spent on the aforementioned products and services designed to treat plantar fasciitis, in addition to millions of visits to both primary care physicians and foot specialists, you might think that the number of people suffering with plantar fasciitis would be decreasing. But rather, it's the opposite. Which begs the question: why?

Answers vary.

Some scholars suggest that it's because of increasing rates of obesity which is a problem because excess weight puts added stress on the plantar fascia.

Others argue that plantar fasciitis is becoming increasingly common as a result of more sedentary lifestyles and a lack of exercise. For instance, with advances in technology and mechanization, certain tasks and jobs now require decreased levels of physical exertion. Spending increased levels of time sitting down in front of a computer or on one's phone has also become more common. Similarly, working from home has become more commonplace, and as a result, many people spend less time on their feet or regularly moving around during the day. With an inactive sedentary lifestyle, the calf muscles, soleus muscles, Achilles tendons, and plantar fascia can shorten and tighten which reduce mobility of the ankles. Then when one engages in activity, the muscles and joints cannot adapt quickly enough to the increased need to be longer and more flexible resulting in strain that goes into the plantar fascia (more to come on this subject in the next chapter).

Conversely, while a lack of exercise can be harmful, so, too, can doing too much physical activity. Increasing physical activity too quickly doesn't give the body enough time to adapt. While the body generally responds to stress by strengthening muscles, bones and tendons, an overload or sudden increase in volume or activity can result in strain. Interestingly, some people find that their foot/feet pain decreases during exercise but greatly increases afterwards. Certain physical activities in particular such as long-distance running, repeated jumping, and dancing place a lot of stress on the heel and attached tissue since during these types of activities your body has to support a load that is several times your bodyweight which can exert a lot of force on your muscles. Still, even doing too much walking can cause strain if the body is not accustomed to a particular workload, perhaps especially if a person is carrying a lot of excess weight and/or uses improper technique, which brings us to the next possible risk factor for plantar fasciitis – foot mechanics.

Foot mechanics are believed to play a part in some cases. That is to say, flat feet, a high arch, inward rolling of the feet, or simply an unusual pattern of walking possibly due to conditions or injuries of the knees or hips can affect the way one's bodyweight is distributed when standing or moving, resulting in extra stress on the plantar fascia.

Just as physical activities can lead to plantar fasciitis, so too can occupations that involve people spending most of their work hours standing or walking, especially on hard surfaces

Wearing improper footwear can further increase the risks. For instance, regularly wearing high heels or flip flops could increase the risk of plantar fasciitis since these types of footwear tend to distribute bodyweight unevenly and do not provide sufficient support for your feet.

Seemingly, age is a factor as well, with plantar fasciitis most common in people between the ages of 40 and 60, though those over 60 or under 40 can certainly still be affected with the condition. Indeed, I've met many people between the ages of 18 and 34 who regularly jump rope and have experienced plantar fasciitis.

So, the risk factors for plantar fasciitis are many and at times seem contradictory.

Free from Plantar Fasciitis Forever

Muscle Chains

It is not recommended to ignore plantar fasciitis since it can not only greatly hinder your lifestyle and regular activities, but if left untreated it could potentially change the way you walk in order to try to avoid or reduce plantar fasciitis pain, which could lead to further problems of the feet, knees, hips, and even back. That is to say, pain in one area of the body could actually be caused by an injury in a completely different region of the body. Take me for example: initially I suffered with pain in only my right foot and heel, and this pain appeared gradually and worsened over time. Then the pain appeared in my left foot and heel as well. Soon thereafter, I experienced some lower back pain.

Given my abovementioned example, it is interesting to note that I've read that in many medical practices, the number of people visiting with complaints of foot and heel pain is similar to those who suffer from lower back pain, which means that many more people could be suffering from plantar fasciitis, since lower back pain could be the result of plantar fasciitis.

You see, this is how muscle chains can work. There are

over 600 muscles in the human body. They are connected into several muscle chains that are a network of muscles, tendons, ligaments, and fascia that work together to enable movement, strength, and stability. Therefore, a particular muscle chain will be involved in producing a particular movement. For instance, the gluteal muscles (commonly known as the butt or bum) and thigh muscles work together in a coordinated manner to perform a squat.

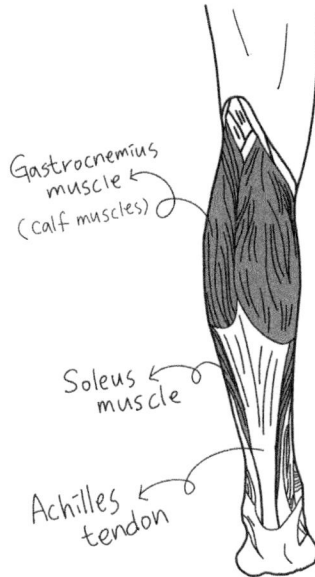

So, while you may be experiencing pain in your foot and heel, or perhaps elsewhere in your body, the source of that pain could be originating from a different area of your body. Tight calves and weak soleus muscles, for example, could cause downward tension through the Achilles tendons which then place the plantar fascia under strain. Tight calf muscles could also cause upwards tension causing issues in the hamstrings or even lower back. One muscle pulls on another muscle affecting another muscle or area of the body like the links in a chain.

While there are many risk factors for plantar fasciitis, it is ultimately caused by strain or wear and tear of the plantar fascia. From my research, together with personal experience, it seems that, one of the most common causes of this strain is the effects of a particular activity such as excess running or jumping combined with a lack of flexibility in the calf muscles and Achilles tendons.

Let's return, for a moment, to one of the aforementioned risk factors for plantar fasciitis, a sedentary lifestyle. When a person is seated, as I am now with my legs up on a couch, my knees are bent and my toes are pointed down which results in a shortening of the calf muscles which then pull on and tighten the Achilles tendons which use the heel bones to pull on the plantar fascia. If the calf muscles are regularly shortened and tight, the plantar fascia is under strain.

Ultimately, what eliminated my plantar fasciitis was implementing particular stretches of the muscles of the lower legs to reduce tightness together with an exercise to strengthen the toes and plantar fascia. These were done several times throughout the day, some at particular times of the day, and in the case of the stretches they were held for longer durations than what is commonly recommended when stretching.

At this point though, it would be remiss of me not to recommend visiting your health care provider to examine your foot and heel pain to rule out causes such as heel spurs, a pinched nerve near the heel, thinning of the heel pad, stress fractures, or Achilles tendonitis.

If your pain is determined to be plantar fasciitis, the great news is that I eventually discovered that it is easy to treat, at least for me and for the many others who made the personal decision to try my protocol.

As a keen jump roper, runner, hiker, and all-around fitness and adventure enthusiast, I've communicated with numerous people who complained of what sounded like plantar fasciitis. I shared with them what worked for me. Those that decided to implement what worked so well for me also experienced the same positive results. I hope you will, too.

My Case Report

I'm approaching 42 years of age. I remain lean, strong, and agile. Throughout my life, I've enjoyed physical pursuits. For instance, I've paraglided in Switzerland, kayaked in Croatia, mountain climbed in Canada, danced in Korea, completed ultra-marathons, and competed in numerous sports including ice and roller hockey, boxing, baseball, rugby, and soccer.

Perhaps it's not surprising then that I've experienced my share of bumps, bruises, stitches, sprains, and fractures.

One of my longest layoffs from physical activity came as a result of an ice hockey-related injury which sidelined me for several months. I broke my big toe, right foot, and ruptured my Achilles tendon.

But, it was my case of plantar fasciitis that had the largest ever impact on my mobility and level of physical activity.

Let's rewind for a moment to mid-June of 2022. That's when I had just finished a 437 kilometer trek which included various types of terrain from flat to hilly and a range of surfaces including concrete, grass, sand, rocks, and dirt.

While trekking, I wore a pair of athletic trail shoes.

During this time, in addition to trekking, I regularly ran barefoot on beaches, rollerbladed, skateboarded, swam in the sea, surfed, jumped rope, and engaged in calisthenics. My footwear varied greatly from wearing nothing to flip flops, aqua shoes, sneakers, boxing boots, and skateboarding shoes.

Living such a physically active lifestyle was nothing new, nor was I not used to regularly wearing different footwear. But, perhaps this time it caught up with me.

Along the final few trails of the trek, I sometimes felt a shooting pain on the bottom of my right foot that continued towards the heel and up through my Achilles tendon and calf muscle. That was the start of my plantar fasciitis.

Over the next 4 weeks, there was often a dull pain in the arch and heel of my right foot. During this time, I abstained from most forms of physical activity except walking and swimming.

Then one day in mid to late July, during an intense jump rope session by the sea, the shooting pain returned. I should have stopped jumping rope, but I was having so much fun and the setting was perfect; waves were crashing on rocks near the shore on a beautiful warm day filled with sunshine and clear blue skies.

I continued jumping rope despite the pain. Silly, I know, but pushing through pain was something I had almost become accustomed to; for a short laundry list of times when I pushed through the 'pain cave', as elite endurance runner Courtney Dauwalter would call it: I played hockey for several weeks with a broken big toe, hiked with a cracked rib, played rugby with stitches in my mouth, ran a marathon with a groin sprain, and took part in a boxing tournament when I had massive blisters on the bottom of each big toe that hindered movement.

However, in more recent years, I had learned to better listen to my body and would rest when deemed necessary. I knew that, without allowing for adequate rest and recovery, doing an activity too often, especially if the activity was done intensely and/or for long durations, could result in pain or injury. But on that bright sunny day by the sea, I didn't heed my body's warning.

At the end of that jump rope session, I could hardly walk. I was just a short 300 meter stroll away from our accommodation, but it took me 20 minutes as I moved at a snail's pace interspersed with many periods of sitting on the ground.

The arch of my right foot was where I felt the most pain. However, since I had experienced pain in the arch of my feet at various times throughout my life as a result of overexertion from sports, I was not overly concerned despite the pain.

I figured that some stretching together with the **RICE** approach for acute injuries would resolve the issue: **R**est, **I**ce, **C**ompression, and **E**levation.

So, for the next two weeks, I avoided any strenuous physical activity. When I had to walk, I sauntered, walking slowly and with gentle footsteps. This, together with ice, compression, and elevation had a positive effect as the pain was beginning to subside. One more week of recovery and I would be okay, I thought.

Indeed, soon thereafter I no longer felt pain in the arch of my right foot.

At that point, I was eager to jump rope again. So, I put on my exercise clothes and with my jump ropes in hand, I made my way out the door to the same location by the sea where I had last jumped rope.

I warmed-up and loosened my body with some mobility movements. Then I eased into the session, beginning at a low intensity and stopping every few minutes. Once I increased the intensity and performed more demanding jump rope moves, I felt a familiar sharp stabbing pain in the arch of my right foot, only this time it was worse.

I stopped jumping rope, sat down, and massaged the area of pain. Then, since I was next to the sea, I decided to submerge my foot under water for some immediate cold therapy. And before attempting to stand and walk, I again massaged my foot and did some rotations of my ankle. However, upon my first steps, the pain was quite severe, not only in the arch of my right foot but also around my heel and Achilles tendon.

I remember thinking, at best, I had just aggravated the previous injury, and at worst, I may have torn something. If you recall, I once broke my right foot and ruptured my Achilles, so I was concerned that I may have done some serious damage.

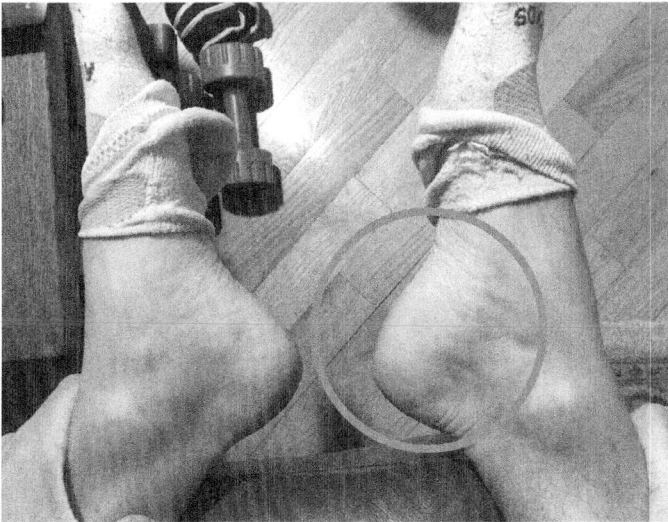

Over the next few days, there was visible swelling of the arch and heel of my right foot (see the image above). My Achilles was also sore, and I had some tenderness in the muscles of my right lower leg. Furthermore, when I stood and walked, it was apparent to my family and friends that I was in discomfort.

Except for walking, I avoided physical activity for the next two weeks, at which point I was relieved that my right lower leg felt relatively fine and my foot was no longer swollen. However, there was pain from the base of my toes to my heel and at the insertion point of my Achilles on the posterior or rear surface of the heel bone, particularly on the first step out of bed in the mornings and after prolonged periods of sitting.

Cold and heat therapy, massage using my hands and a ball, compression, elevation, stretching, and the application of an anti-inflammatory ointment did nothing to relieve this pain.

I searched the internet for answers. All signs indicated that I was suffering from plantar fasciitis. A conversation with a friend of mine who is a doctor supported this view.

I was informed that it was not uncommon for people to suffer from plantar fasciitis for several months, some even several years. That was disconcerting. But, given that I was healthy, relatively young, and tended to recover well from injuries, I thought I could recover quite quickly.

I began following instructions to facilitate recovery. This essentially meant limiting cardio to necessary walking and riding a stationary bike, more massaging of the feet and lower legs, and performing plantar fasciitis exercises.

In the next section, I will provide details about the plantar fasciitis exercises since the information and movements could be of benefit to others depending on their injury. However, I received little benefit or reduction in my plantar fasciitis pain following this approach. But, again, that doesn't mean this approach or the exercises don't have merit. For instance, I've done some of the exercises long before I ever heard of plantar fasciitis and will likely continue to do them on occasion because I think they provide benefits not limited to plantar fasciitis treatment. Yet, in terms of my case of plantar fasciitis, they did little to relieve my pain.

Free from Plantar Fasciitis Forever

Common Plantar Fasciitis Exercises

Toe Extensions

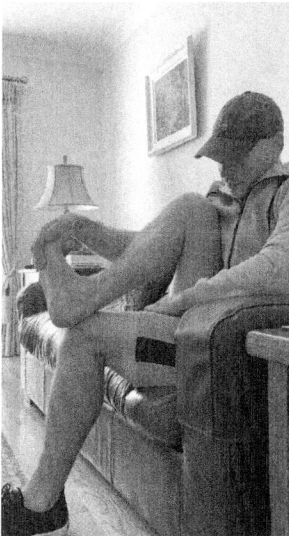

Step 1: While sitting, cross the affected leg/foot over the other leg or rest the affected leg/foot on a chair or sofa.

Step 2: Bend the affected foot upwards as far as possible towards your knee.

Step 3: Using one hand, grasp the toes of the affected foot and bend them as much as possible towards your knee. You will feel a stretch along the plantar fascia.

Step 4: Hold the stretch for 10 seconds. Then rest a few seconds before repeating the stretch.

▶ Do 6 sets for a total stretching time of 1 minute. Do this drill 3 times a day for a total stretching time of 3 minutes.

Optional: Using your other hand, massage the plantar fascia while it is being stretched.

* If you have pain in both feet and heels, perform the above exercise for both feet.

Towel Curls

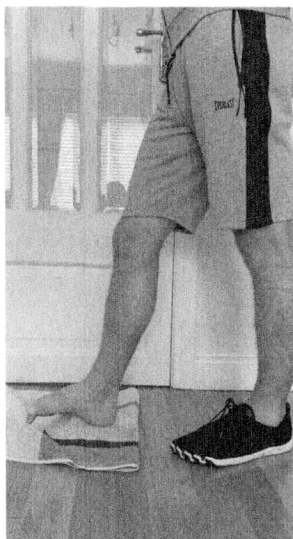

Step 1: Place a small towel on the floor.

Step 2: While standing or sitting, place only your affected foot on the towel.

Step 3: Using only your toes, scrunch the towel towards you by curling your toes.

Step 4: Then, using only your toes, push the towel away from you by uncurling or straightening your toes.

▶ Repeat 10 times. Do this drill 2 times a day, once in the morning and once in the afternoon or evening.

Optional: To make this exercise more challenging, place a light weight or weighted object like a book or tin of soup on the end of the towel in front of your foot.

* If you have pain in both feet and heels, perform the above exercise for both feet.

Towel Stretch

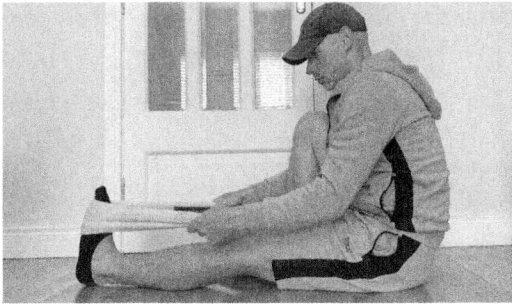

Step 1: While sitting and resting your legs straight out in front of you on your bed, floor, or sofa, place a towel around your foot just under your toes.

Step 2: Holding the ends of the towel in your hands, gently pull back the ends of the towel towards you so that your foot stretches towards you. You should feel a stretch in your calf muscles.

▶ Hold the stretch for 30 seconds. Rest for a few seconds before repeating the exercise. Do this 3 times for a total stretching time of 90 seconds. Perform this drill once or twice per day.

* If you have pain in both feet and heels, perform the above exercise for both feet.

Wall Calf Stretch

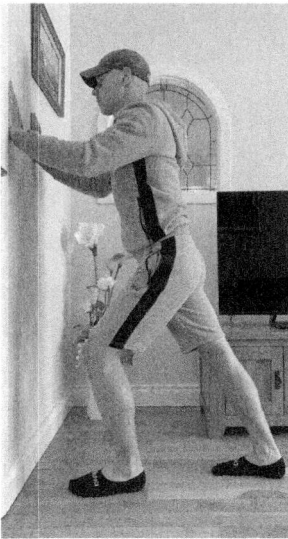

Step 1: Facing a wall, stand about 3 feet away from the wall.

Step 2: Place both hands on the wall for support while simultaneously taking a large step forward with your unaffected foot. Your affected or injured foot should be in the rear. Your front leg should be bent at the knee while your back leg should be kept straight. Keep both feet pointing straight ahead.

Step 3: Gently shift your bodyweight forward while making sure to keep the heel of your affected foot on the ground. You should feel a stretch in the calf muscle of your back leg.

▶ Hold this stretch for 30 seconds. Rest a few seconds before repeating. Do this 3 times for a total stretching time of 90 seconds. Repeat this drill 3 times per day.

* If you have pain in both feet and heels, perform the above exercise for both feet.

Wall Soleus Stretch

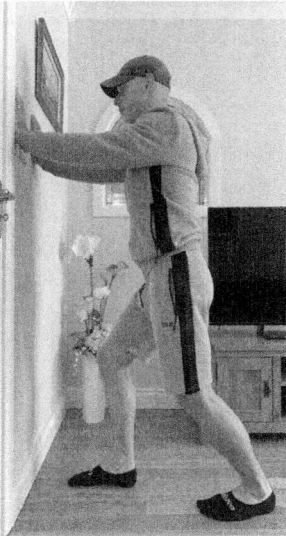

Step 1: Facing a wall, stand about 3 feet away from the wall.

Step 2: Place both hands on the wall for support while simultaneously taking a large step forward with your unaffected foot. Your affected or injured foot should be in the rear. Your front leg should be bent at the knee and your back leg should also be bent slightly to isolate the soleus muscle. Keep both feet on the floor and pointing straight ahead.

Step 3: Gently shift your bodyweight forward while making sure to keep the heel of your affected foot on the ground. You should feel a stretch in the lower part of your back leg.

▶ Hold this stretch for 30 seconds. Rest a few seconds before repeating. Do this 3 times for a total stretching time of 90 seconds. Repeat this drill 3 times per day.

* If you have pain in both feet and heels, perform the above exercise for both feet.

In addition to the above exercises, as previously mentioned, I limited my cardio to walking plus using a stationary bicycle. I also regularly massaged my feet and lower legs with a combination of my hands, a small massage ball or rolling pin. If I were in pain after walking, I sometimes applied an ice pack to the bottom of my foot or submerged my foot in an ice bath. Furthermore, I regularly applied an anti-inflammatory ointment.

Injury Update & Onset of Bilateral Plantar Fasciitis

8 weeks later and I still had not recovered.

For someone who thoroughly enjoys exercise and being physically active in the outdoors, it was a tough time. Not only have I always enjoyed challenging myself physically, but I also reap mood-altering benefits from exercise especially moderate to intense cardiovascular activity.

I must note that, while I couldn't do cardio to boost my energy levels or mood when necessary, I still engaged in resistance training since I have long known the benefits and importance of maintaining muscle and strength. So, a few times a week, I did some resistance training for my upper body as well as for my legs using movements that wouldn't impact my injured foot. Similarly, when my foot was in a cast a number of years ago, I still regularly did weight training or calisthenics for my upper body and good leg. Again, I believe that maintaining muscle and strength is vital even if it means working around an injury.

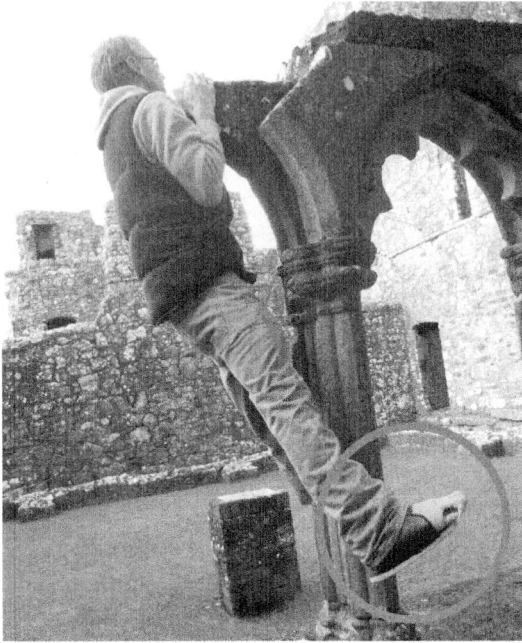

With previous injuries of mine, there was generally an obvious outward sign of injury such as bruising, stitches, a splint, cast, or crutches. But, with plantar fasciitis, this is not the case.

Friends and family members were not accustomed to me being so inactive and found it somewhat strange that I had not made a more rapid recovery especially from something as 'minor' as an injury which was not even visible to the eye.

And worse was still to come.

Not only was I experiencing pain in my right foot, but my

left foot and heel had begun to bother me as well.

Given that I couldn't use my right foot to support my bodyweight as I normally would when standing and walking, I must have inadvertently altered my gait and posture, that is, how I stood and walked. Therefore, my left leg and foot would have had to compensate and continually bear more workload. As a result, pain and injury eventually ensued.

I now had bilateral plantar fasciitis, that is, pain in the bottom of both feet and heels.

At that point, it seemed like plantar fasciitis was perhaps something I might just have to learn to live with, as many others were seemingly doing, having read so many stories about others whose plantar fasciitis impeded their day-to-day lives for years without resolve.

So, what did I do? Almost out of frustration, I tried jumping rope, and of course, it was painful.

Also, a week later, when it came time to meet my nieces who I hadn't seen in two years, I didn't want to avoid play because of plantar fasciitis. And so, when I noticed a few jump ropes scattered in their yard, despite being in pain, I demonstrated some advanced jump rope moves. But once I stopped, it was as if I had just poured gasoline over the fire which was my feet. I was in extreme pain but tried in earnest to remain a stoic uncle.

Several more months had passed and still no progress regarding my case of plantar fasciitis. At least, though, it was winter, which meant it was less enticing to spend time outdoors between the cold, rain, and less hours of daylight.

Then, one evening, while watching an old YouTube video of mine where I performed the middle splits, I had a lightbulb moment of sorts.

Light-Bulb Moment (Strengthening and 2 Minute Stretch Holds)

When I initially began learning the middle splits, I did what many were advised to do, hold the various stretches for 20-30 seconds. However, it was only when I held the stretches for much longer durations that I made progress. Instead of holding stretches for half a minute, I held each stretch for 2 minutes, so I was amassing far more stretching time in any given day. This was something I learned from strength coach Pavel Tsatsouline during one of his interviews with Tim Ferriss when they were discussing how to do the splits.

So, that's when I decided that I would hold the aforementioned plantar fasciitis stretches[1] for much longer durations.

---

1 Toe Extensions, Towel Stretch, Wall Calf Stretch, Wall Soleus Stretch

I did this for a few weeks, but the improvements were uninspiring.

However, I believe that, for many people suffering with plantar fasciitis, holding the aforementioned stretches for 2 minutes a few times per day for 1-3 weeks could eliminate their plantar fasciitis. This optimistic opinion is supported by feedback from hundreds of viewers in the comments section of a video I came across around that time on YouTube about treating plantar fasciitis by former professional triathlete Brad Kearns, who eliminated his plantar fasciitis by holding similar stretches for 2 minutes (I encourage you to check out Brad Kearns' YouTube channel for lots of great health and fitness information).

Why wasn't I having the same results? I remember thinking my case of plantar fasciitis must have been so stubborn due to aggravation from excess physical activity including jumping rope in addition to being connected with my previous ice hockey-related foot and Achilles tendon injury.

That's when I had a second light bulb moment.

During Pavel Tsatsouline's interview with Tim Ferriss, he talked about the importance of including an element of strength training when learning the middle splits, and so, that's what I did en route to learning how to successfully do the middle splits. That is to say, not only did I hold middle split stretches for long durations, but I also included some resistance when doing certain stretching exercises.

Aha! Maybe that was one of the missing keys in terms of treating my plantar fasciitis. So, I decided to include a strengthening exercise in my protocol.

Furthermore, I recalled that, as kid, there were two lower leg stretches that we often did after soccer practices and games which I had not yet tried. So, I decided that I would try those two stretches and hold them for 2 minutes.

And, in just one day of implementing the strengthening exercise and the two stretches, I experienced some immediate relief.

After having suffered for so many months, it was almost astonishing that within just a few days of implementing this new protocol, my feet and heel pain were decreasing substantially, so much so that I believed I would be ready in time to participate in a St. Patrick's Day half-marathon that was less than three weeks away.

Inspired by the noticeable improvements and the growing possibility of being able to take part in a running event with a large group of people to raise money for a good cause filled me with enthusiasm, and so I stepped up my plantar fasciitis treatment protocol in earnest.

In the next section, I will share exactly what I did to completely eliminate my plantar fasciitis in two weeks.

Perhaps best of all, the protocol involves no plantar fasciitis products or services and can be done from the comfort of your home.

Let's get started!

Free from Plantar Fasciitis Forever

My Plantar Fasciitis Recovery Protocol

Recall that plantar fasciitis is, for many people, very painful with the first steps of the day, so I took action each morning before even placing my feet on the ground. I did two things: (1) a simple, very brief massage of the arch of my feet to help release stress and tension and to warm-up the area, and (2) Ankle Circles aka Ankle Rotations in order to open up and stretch the tendons and ligaments of my ankle joints as well as gently loosen the feet and calves.

Arch Massage

Since I had pain in both feet and heels, I performed this for both feet, one at a time. Using both hands, although you could use just one hand, I applied downward pressure with my thumbs on top of my foot, and upward pressure with my fingers on the arch of my foot, moving up and down the plantar fascia. I did this for about 20 seconds on each foot. Then I rubbed the plantar fascia for just 5-10 seconds to further warm the area.

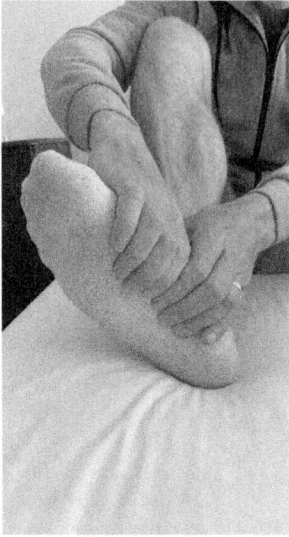

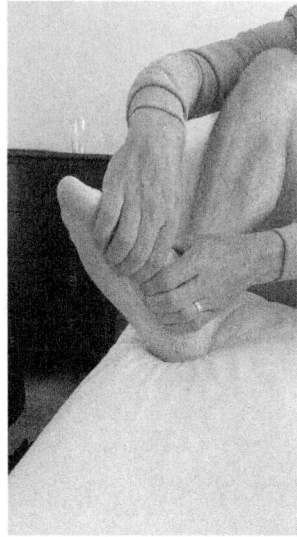

Ankle Circles aka Ankle Rotations

I performed these while lying down in bed, but I could have also done them while sitting on my bed with my legs hanging over the side of the bed.

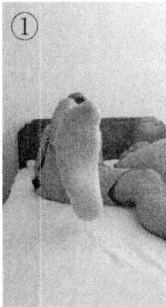

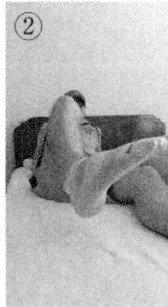

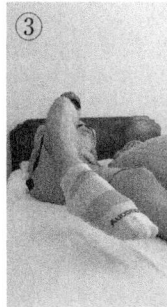

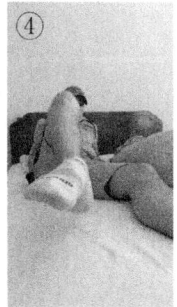

While lying down, I bent my knee and raised my foot a few inches off the bed. Next, as the name of the exercise implies, I made circles with my ankles. Beginning with my right foot, I rotated my foot anticlockwise for 10-15

rotations. Then I did 10-15 clockwise rotations. I repeated this for my left foot. Because my ankles are fairly flexible, I began with large ankle circles to open up my ankle joints. But you can start with smaller circles and gradually increase the diameter of your rotations. If you feel any discomfort or pain, begin with smaller circles.

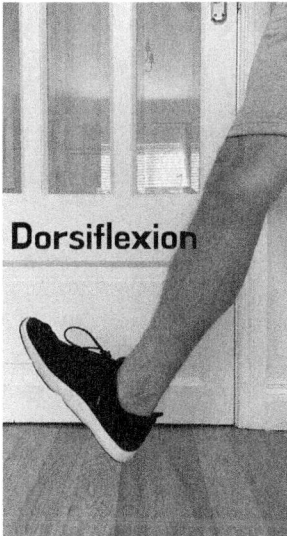

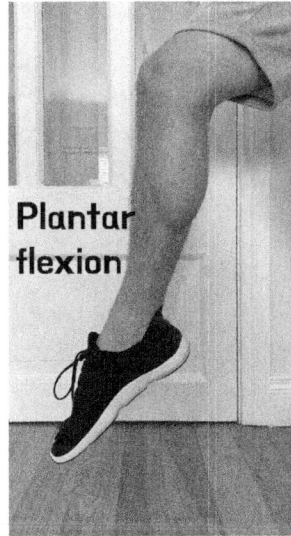

* I believe that Ankle Circles are a great movement to do after prolonged periods of sitting or lying down, whether or not you have plantar fasciitis.

After briefly massaging my feet and doing ankle circles, it was time to place my feet on the ground. But again, since the first steps of the day after sleeping can be extremely painful, I didn't immediately start walking after getting out of bed. Instead, after placing my feet on the ground, I did an exercise for strengthening the toes and plantar fascia as well as for gently engaging the muscles of the lower legs. I believe this exercise, which we'll refer to as the Forward Lean, was vital for recovery. In fact, every time after performing this exercise, my feet felt much better than they did just beforehand.

Forward Lean

After placing both feet on the ground, stand up. You may have to use your hands and arms for assistance to go from seated to standing.

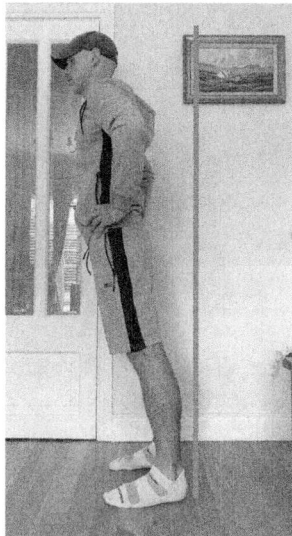

A word first about safety when performing this exercise: Ideally, when you stand up, you could be facing a wall, with your body about 3 feet from the wall. If you can't face a wall, a sturdy bedroom dresser, drawer, or wardrobe can work, too. These are not necessary, but they can help perform the exercise in a safer manner. So, worse case, you may have to take a step or two so that you are facing a wall about 3 feet away. Of course, if you have confidence in your ability not to fall, you don't necessarily need to use a wall or other sturdy object for support. If in any doubt about your safety, you can even do this exercise while placing your hands on a sturdy object for support throughout the exercise, but the key is to engage the feet, not lower or raise your body with your hands and arms.

Okay, now that you're standing, keep your hips, shoulder, and head in a straight line, and stand with your arms at your sides, crossed in front of your body, or resting on your hips. Maintain this posture as you very slowly lean forward, leaning at the ankles and letting the rest of the body follow. By leaning forward, you are shifting your bodyweight on to your toes, and therefore you will notice immediately that your toes, especially your big toes, push down into the floor. You will be pushing your toes into the floor with more force the more you lean forward. Slowly lean forward to the point where you feel like you could fall if you were not aggressively pushing your toes into the floor. Try to hold this position for 5 seconds before pushing your body back to a vertical or upright position by pressing down forcefully with your toes. That's one repetition. Repeat this 5 times.

Almost any time I stood up from a seated position, I did at least one repetition of the Forward Lean and sometimes two to five repetitions. I also did two to three repetitions of the Forward Lean exercise just before going to bed.

Do the Forward Lean without wearing shoes — either barefoot or wearing socks — at least a few times throughout the day, such as in the morning, in the evening, and before bed. It's okay to do the Forward Lean while wearing shoes, but you might find that the sensation and engagement of the toes and plantar fascia is slightly different than without shoes.

Perhaps this is too much information, but some of the males with whom I shared this protocol did the Forward Lean in the bathroom while standing over the toilet or urinal. In other words, they incorporated the Forward Lean throughout their day in convenient ways. You could, for instance, do the Forward Lean while waiting for the kettle to boil and use a countertop for support if necessary. Similarly, before or after brushing your teeth, you could do the Forward Lean.

I would have probably performed the Forward Lean exercise close to 20 times in any given day. And although my feet are fine now, I still do the Forward Lean a few times throughout the day. One, it feels good, and two, there is a proven connection between falling and weak toes and feet. So, simply doing this exercise could go a long way to helping avoid falls now or later in life. Falls are a leading cause of injury and even injury-related death among older adults.

The Forward Lean exercise is beneficial whether you have pain in one or both feet and heels.

Once I had completed several repetitions of the Forward Lean exercise after getting out of bed, then I soon completed the next key exercise, which I will refer to as the Step Stretch.

So, each morning, after completing the Forward Lean exercise, I headed outside and made my way to a concrete curb; technically, before heading outside I used the bathroom and also drank water to hydrate. You don't need a curb, nor do you need to go outside to perform the Step Stretch, but for close to 15 years, I've enjoyed going outside in the natural light and air soon after rising. Of note, it seems that recent research is finding many benefits of getting natural light exposure in the morning including increased alertness, so if you can do the Step Stretch outside shortly after awakening, you could reap several benefits in addition to working towards relieving your plantar fasciitis.

Step Stretch

For the Step Stretch, you will need an object that is anywhere from 3 to 6 inches high. A smaller 'step' could work best if you have small feet, while a higher step might suit longer feet, though this is not necessarily the case.

For the Step Stretch, I recommend wearing shoes to avoid any abrasions or friction to the feet or heels from rough surfaces. Furthermore, if performing the Step Stretch with both feet at the same time, a smaller step such as 3 to 4 inches high works well, since it's easier to stand with good balance. If performing the Step Stretch one foot at a time, standing with good balance is less of an issue even the step is high, such as 5 to 6 inches.

Which brings me to the next point: The Step Stretch can be performed using only your injured foot or it can be done using both feet at the same time. For the time being, let's assume just your left foot is injured (see Image 1 on the next page). Now, using your left foot, while keeping the heel of your foot on the ground, angle your foot so that the top of the step reaches around the midpoint of the 'ball' of your foot, technically called the metatarsophalangeal joint. The 'ball' is the area of your foot between the toes and the arch. At this point, you will likely feel a stretch in your lower left leg. If not, gently lean forward to cause a different stretching sensation in your lower leg. As you lean forward, try to keep your body relatively straight or in alignment, but it is okay if you need to raise your arms out in front as a type of counterbalance or place your hands on your hips for balance. Using a timer, such as the clock on your phone, hold the stretch for 2 minutes. During this stretch hold, you can gently lean farther forward or adjust your foot on the step to deepen the stretch in your lower leg. For instance, after 30 seconds or so, if you want to deepen the stretch, you could lean farther forward and/or angle your foot so that the top of the step reaches around the bottom of the 'ball' of your foot.

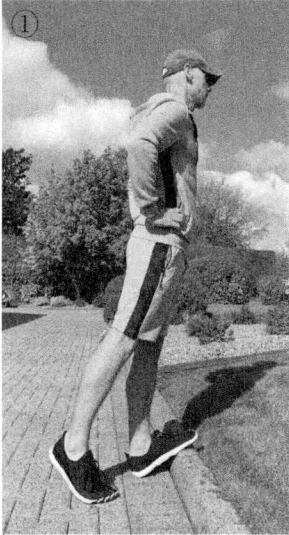

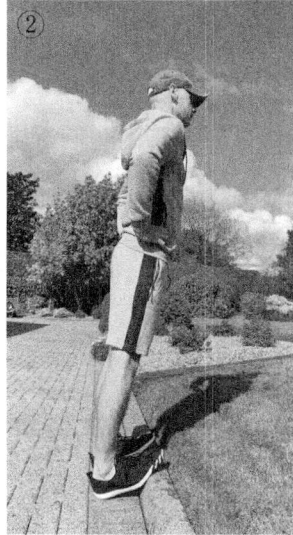

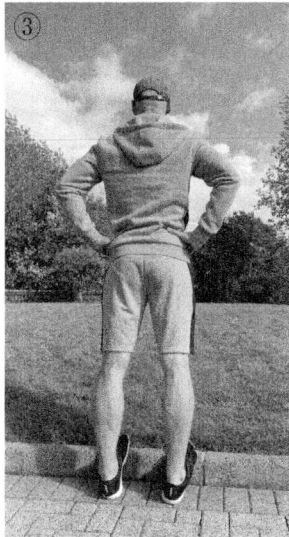

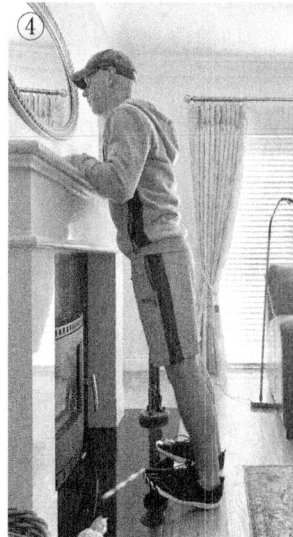

When performing the Step Stretch with just one foot on the step, it's okay and natural if the heel of your other foot comes off the ground as you lean forward (see Image 1 on page 57).

Also, while it's important to straighten your leg or legs that are on the step, you don't have to completely lock out your knee or knees, that is to say, you don't have to press your knee or knees as far back as possible so that there is no bend in the knee. A slight bend in the knee is okay.

If you have plantar fasciitis in both feet, as I did, then you will want to perform the Step Stretch for both feet, either one foot at a time as just described or you can perform it on both feet at the same time (see Images 2, 3, and 4 on page 57). Regardless, begin by first placing one foot on the step and then the other foot.

Many of the people who tried my protocol were amazed at how much better their feet felt after completing even just one round of both the Forward Lean and the Step Stretch. The two exercises are fantastic for strengthening the feet and for stretching the muscles, tendons, and ligaments of the lower legs.

Holding stretches for 2 minutes is likely much longer than you are accustomed to holding stretches and therefore may be a bit uncomfortable at least at first. However, I found that, in terms of treating plantar fasciitis, it was necessary in order to attain relief and a complete reduction in pain. As I said, when learning the middle splits, it was only when I held stretches for 2 minutes and incorporated some strengthening exercises that I began to make steady progress. This same approach worked for eliminating my plantar fasciitis.

I did the Step Stretch 3 to 6 times a day. Each set of the Step Stretch was usually done a few hours apart such as once in the morning, once in the afternoon, and once in the evening. Some days, I did the Step Stretch more frequently; in addition to the above, some days I did it mid-morning, late afternoon, and at night. Whether at home or in public, it was always easy to find sturdy objects which were suitable for the Step Stretch.

I would suggest doing the Step Stretch a minimum of 3 times a day.

We still have one other exercise to discuss, which I refer to as the Wall Foot Stretch.

Wall Foot Stretch

For the Wall Foot Stretch, while you can do it barefoot, I recommend wearing shoes or at the very least socks to avoid any abrasions or friction to the feet or heels from rough surfaces.

With this exercise, as the name suggests, you will use a

wall, though other vertical sturdy surfaces work well such as the jambs of a doorframe or a steel pole. If you have plantar fasciitis in both feet, you will repeat this exercise for the other foot.

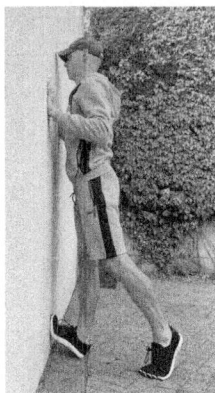

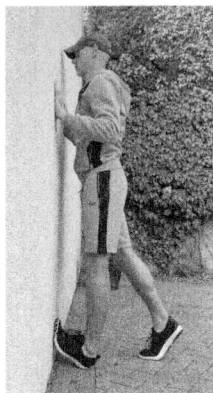

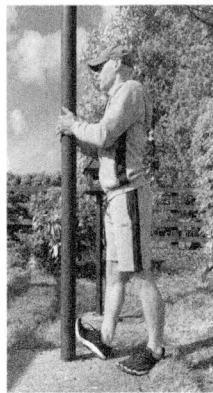

Begin facing the wall about two feet away. Place both hands on the wall. Next, place the bottom of your big toe of your injured foot against the wall; the bottom of your other toes will also touch the wall, which is perfect, but we'll concentrate on the big toe. Keep your heel on the floor or ground. Your heel will be 4 to 8 inches or so away from the wall, depending on the size of your foot. Now, keeping your body straight and using your rear foot as leverage, lean forward while focusing on putting your body weight onto your big toe that is against the wall. You should feel a stretch in the plantar fascia of your injured foot and even up the base of your lower leg. Deepen the stretch by leaning farther forward and/or bending the rear leg. Using a timer, hold the stretch for 2 minutes. You can experiment with the angle between the bottom of your big toe and your heel and how it affects the feel of the stretch. Perhaps you achieve a greater stretch when your heel is closer or farther away from the wall.

Perform the Wall Foot Stretch 3 times a day, such as once in the mornings, afternoons, and evenings. Performing it more than 3 times a day is okay but aim for a minimum of 3 times.

There you are my hopefully soon-to-be-free-from-plantar-fasciitis-friends, those are the key exercises that enabled me to completely eliminate my severe case of bilateral plantar fasciitis in only 14 days.

Once I made a connection between a feat I had previously accomplished — learning the middle splits — and then applying a similar approach to treating my plantar fasciitis, I was able to walk, jump, and run pain free after just two weeks.

For that reason, I felt compelled to write this book. I believe it is one of our duties to share what has healed or helped us, not just in terms of physical injuries but in other areas of our lives. In other words, I believe that we sometimes suffer so that ultimately we can help others avoid similar suffering. To overcome plantar fasciitis and not share my solution with others would be a waste of a painful learning experience.

Free from Plantar Fasciitis Forever

Addendum and Additional Exercises for Foot and Lower Leg Health

It has been six months since I eliminated my plantar fasciitis. And, given the physical activities I regularly perform, some people might think I'm trying to make my feet and heel pain return.

As previously stated, as soon as I recovered, I completed a half-marathon. I felt so relieved to be pain-free that I would have done a full-marathon if it were available. And since then, I have ran, biked, mountain climbed, swam, boxed, did acrobatics, martial arts, and of course, jumped rope intensely (in case you don't know, I have a jump rope YouTube channel with jump rope tutorials, workouts, and challenges. For more details, please visit my channel: https://www.youtube.com/c/TheWayoftheJumpRope).

To prevent plantar fasciitis and/or to prevent it from returning, I recommend doing the exercises included in my protocol a few times throughout the week. Indeed, I still do them. However, I do far fewer repetitions or sets. For example, I do the Forward Lean whenever I feel like it, which usually happens to be at least once or several times throughout the day because I believe it's great for foot and leg health, plus I now just enjoy doing it since my feet always feel good afterwards. The same goes for the Step Stretch; I usually do it once a day, sometimes twice, such as once in the morning and maybe again in the evening. I do the Wall Foot Stretch a few times a week, typically as part of my 'cooldown' after an intense jump rope session or other form of leg intensive cardio.

Five additional exercises that I regularly do and did long before my case of plantar fasciitis for foot and leg health are seated soleus raises, calf raises, toe sitting, foot tapping, and toe raises.

Calf Raises

The gastrocnemius, more commonly known as the calf muscles or calves, are far more than just large, powerful, eye-catching muscles that are easy to see while wearing shorts. They support you when you stand and allow you to move your feet and lower legs. Without the calves, we couldn't walk, run, jump, rotate our ankles, or even flex our feet. With each step we take, they help absorb our bodyweight and minimize impact. Despite their importance, calf muscles are often neglected when it comes to training. Fortunately, they are an easy muscle group to target.

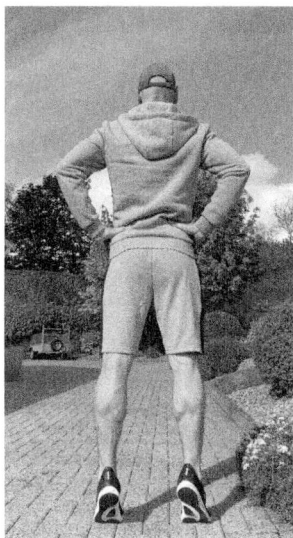

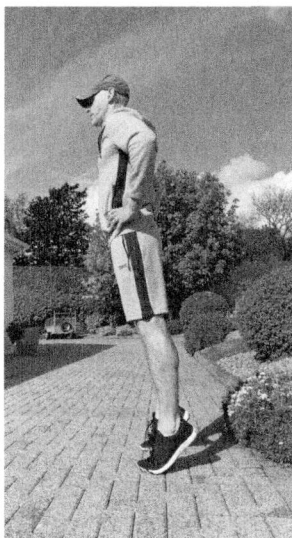

A terrific exercise to target the calf muscles is the standing calf raise which can be performed virtually anywhere.

To perform the basic standing calf raise, begin by standing on the floor with your feet about shoulder-width-apart or even a bit closer together. Keep your toes pointing forward. Your legs should be straight but a slight bend in your knees is okay. Keep your upper body straight. You can keep your arms at the sides of your body, crossed in front of your body, or resting on your hips. Next, slowly raise your heels as high as you can off the floor while keeping your toes on the floor. To raise your heels off the floor, the toes and balls of your feet will press downwards into the floor. When you're standing as much on the tips of your toes as possible, pause for one or two seconds, squeezing the calf muscles. Then slowly lower your heels back to the floor. That's one repetition. Work your way up to the point where you can perform 20-25 repetitions in a row. You could do 2 to 3 sets per week. However, if your calves are fairly small and weak, you could do a few sets several days a week, such as 2 to 3 sets on Mondays, Wednesdays, and Fridays. To make the movement more challenging, you could hold weights in your hands at the sides of your body or you could wear a weighted vest or a rucksack with heavy objects or weights inside.

For more variations of the calf raise plus calf muscle workouts, refer to this playlist: https://www.youtube.com/playlist?list=PLZ-WVpIl4S5iirGRJF27c8zxiqnHRPwMn

Seated Soleus Raises

Unlike calf muscles, soleus muscles are less prominent and harder to see as they are located underneath the calves and attach to the heel via the Achilles tendon. Yet, they are extremely important when it comes to performing simple every day activities like standing and walking as well as running, dancing, and jumping.

Strong soleus muscles mean greater stability, and therefore better balance and a lesser chance of falling. They also assist with blood flow to the heart, increasing the flow of oxygen and nutrients throughout the body which has an influence on well-being and physical performance.

On the other hand, weak soleus muscles will more easily fatigue and strain the calf muscles.

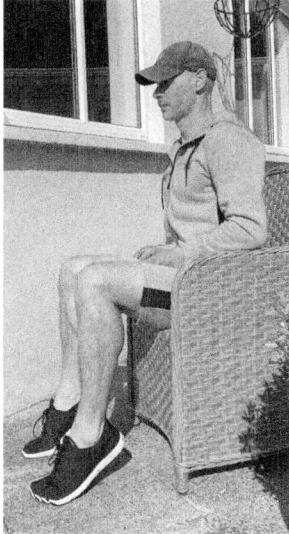

While the soleus muscles are often ignored in training programs, doing a few sets of seated soleus raises throughout the week may greatly help reduce your risk of lower leg injury and increase your performance and mobility. And since the exercise requires that you sit down, it's a convenient exercise to incorporate into your day.

Seated soleus raises are similar to calf raises except they are done while seated with your knees bent at a 90 degree angle. Keep your upper body straight. Your feet should start flat on the floor. Raise your heels as high as you can off the floor while keeping the toes and balls of your feet on the floor. Then lower your heels back to the floor. That's one repetition. You could work your way up to doing 20 repetitions 2-3 times a week.

To make the exercise more challenging, you could add some resistance by simply pressing downwards just above your knees using your hands. Begin gently and increase downwards pressure depending on how you feel. Or, you could place weights or a weighted object on your thighs.

Toe Sitting

Toe sitting is great for ankle and toe mobility, though it can be challenging and somewhat painful if you are new to the movement.

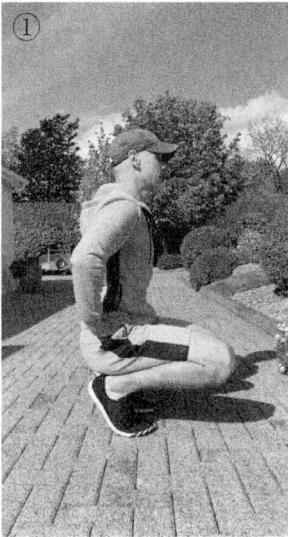

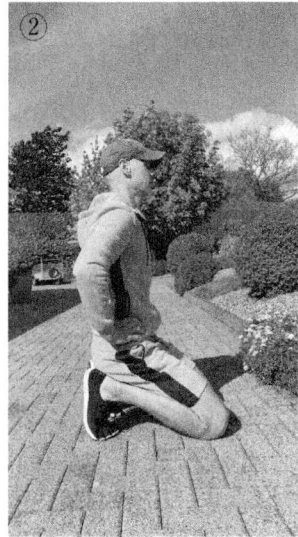

To perform toe sitting, bend your knees and lower your body down towards the floor while simultaneously raising your heels off the floor. At this point, you will be in a squat-like position with your body weight largely supported by the toes and balls of your feet (see Image 1 on page 68). Next, slowly move your upper body forward as you gently bring your knees to the ground (see Image 2 on page 68). If you decide to try this movement, you might only be able to maintain the Toe Sitting position for a few seconds before experiencing some tightness or low level pain in your toes, feet, or lower legs. With practice and patience, you may be able to work your way to the point where you can comfortably sit in this position for 1 to 2 minutes.

Foot Tapping

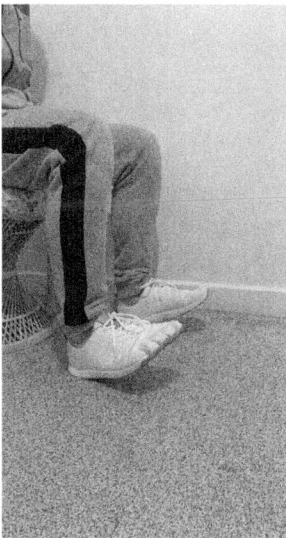

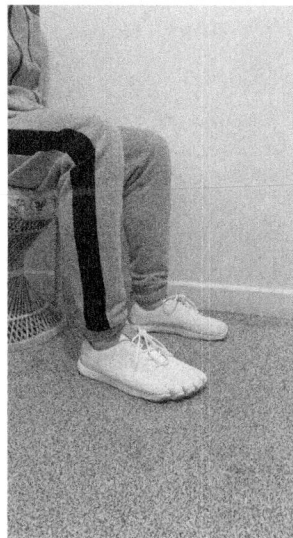

Foot tapping is a simple and effective way to strengthen the tibialis anterior muscle which runs alongside the tibia, also known as the shinbone. Foot tapping can be performed from a standing or seated position. If you do them while standing, you may need to hold onto a sturdy object for balance. To perform foot tapping, keep the heel of your feet on the ground. Then raise the rest of your foot off the ground a few inches before lowering your foot and tapping it against the ground. That's one repetition. You can do foot tapping with one foot at a time or both feet at the same time. Or you could do them in an alternate fashion, that is, perform one repetition with your right foot then one repetition with your left foot. Work your way up to the point where you can perform 20-25 repetitions for each foot. You could do 2 to 3 sets per week.

Toe Raises

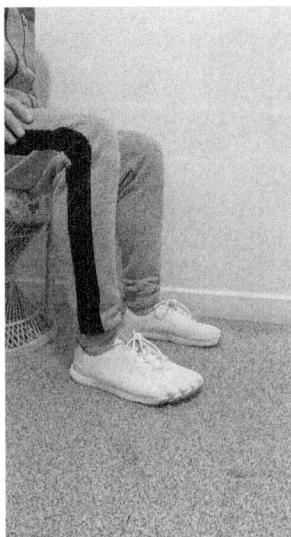 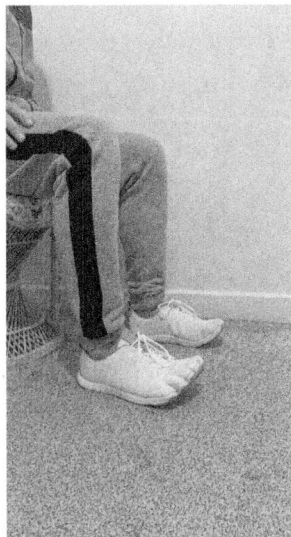

Toe raises can be performed from a standing or seated position. If you do them while standing, you may need to hold onto a sturdy object for balance. To perform toe raises, raise only your toes off the ground, flexing at the balls of your feet. The object of the movement is to raise your toes off the ground while keeping the rest of your foot planted on the ground. Raise your toes and hold for a second before lowering them to the ground. That's one repetition. Work your way up to the point where you can perform 20-25 repetitions for each foot. You could do 2 to 3 sets per week. You can do toe raises with one foot at a time or both feet at the same time. Or you could do them in an alternate fashion, that is, perform one repetition with your right foot then one repetition with your left foot.

Free from Plantar Fasciitis Forever

Conclusion

We've reached the end of the book, but hopefully for you it marks the beginning of living pain-free forever from plantar fasciitis.

I believe you will get some immediate relief the very first day after trying the techniques covered in my protocol.

I suffered for many months with severe foot and heel pain. I wrote this book so you don't have to experience the same torment or waste your valuable time, energy, and money on treatments that deliver poor results.

That's it!

I am purposely keeping this conclusion short because I want you to get started immediately on eliminating your plantar fasciitis.

It's time to swap wincing in pain while you walk with jumping for joy.

About the Author

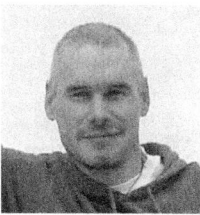

Andrew Dunne is a certified personal trainer, jump rope instructor, teacher, and author whose writing has been published in newspapers, magazines, and academic journals. He writes on subjects including fitness, body image, adolescence, ageing, sport, travel, and adventure. He is the author of Jump Rope Johnny and the Inspiring Mr. P. He grew up in Canada but earned his master's degree in Dublin, Ireland.

As a kid, Andrew excelled in sports and athletics. Far less of his attention and enthusiasm were devoted to schoolwork, which made him a regular in detention and the principal's office. That was until a substitute teacher, whose brother was a professional athlete, pulled him aside and said that if he applied himself in class with the same focus and drive as he did with sports, he could do well academically.

Given the impact his teacher had on his life, perhaps it's not surprising that Andrew later became a teacher, though he will forever try to remain a student, full of curiosity and keen to learn new things. He has busked and tap danced in Korea, paraglided in Switzerland, kayaked in Croatia, competed in boxing, and completed ultra-marathons. He lives with his wife and enjoys starting each day with coffee and reading.

More books by Andrew Dunne

Jump Rope Johnny

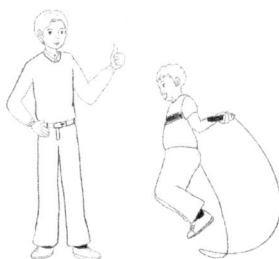

and the Inspiring Mr. P

ANDREW T. DUNNE

An uplifting tale of self-discovery and transformation

Combining wisdom, empathy, hope, and joy, Jump Rope Johnny and the Inspiring Mr. P tells the story of Johnny Peter, a boy struggling with weight issues, bullying, and a lack of self-belief.

Johnny's life is forever changed when he meets Mr. P, a substitute teacher with a passion for jumping rope.

Could the life lessons that Mr. P shares with Johnny also inspire change in your life?

Available from amazon: https://amzn.to/3P3RuAi

Printed in Great Britain
by Amazon

51321735R00046